Surviving the "*Business*" of Healthcare

—*Knowledge is Power!*

*A Unique Perspective from a 4th Generation
Family Practice Provider and Now Cancer Patient*

Barbara Galutia Regis, M.S., PA-C

outskirts
press

Outskirts Press, Inc.
http://www.outskirtspress.com

ISBN: 978-1-4787-6049-8

Library of Congress Control Number: 2018907943

Cover Photo © 2019 www.gettyimages.com. All rights reserved - used with permission.

Outskirts Press and the "OP" logo are trademarks belonging to Outskirts Press, Inc.

PRINTED IN THE UNITED STATES OF AMERICA

For Mom

Your love, support and kindness
will live on forever.

I am proud to be your "kid".

Gratitude starts with your tribe: past and present.

This book is dedicated to my friends, family, and patients who have entrusted me with your care over the years. I am also grateful to my students, as I love teaching and I learned so much from each one of you. I now have a new family, and we are sharing and learning from our melanoma journeys. Together, we will find a cure!

Thanks to my lovely, amazing sister-in-law, Diane Casenta Galutia for your advice and help with editing this book and to Karen Nowicki, my dear friend and president at Phoenix Business Radio X for encouraging me to never give up. Your advice and support have been so helpful!

I am so grateful to my parents, Dave, Rich, Lisa, Bob, Monica, George, May, and my nieces, nephews, and our friends for your continued support as I work through this journey and also advocate for better health.

I am also grateful for close friends: Joe, DeDe, Mike, Deb, Joe, Pam, Linda, and Scott as you have been so important to Tony and me throughout the last several decades.

I also want to thank Mary, Karen W., Usha M., Maria B., April S., and Beth L. (friend and dermatology PA) along with the rest of my dear friends, business partners, and coworkers, past and present. I have learned so much from each of you.

I also owe so much gratitude to our dear Old English Sheepdogs, past and present: Beau, Winnie, and Abby. Your unconditional love has been amazing.

Finally, to the rock and love of my life: my husband Tony. Oh, you have been through a lot, and your patience and support are so appreciated. To many more years together, as I am eternally grateful for you and your strength.

Table of Contents

1. One phone call can change your life and perspective forever 1

2. Helping You Survive the "Business" of Healthcare: Knowledge Is Power! 11

3. Following in My Dad's Footsteps 13

4. Why I Love Being a Primary Care Provider (PCP) 16

5. Why a Physician Assistant (PA)? Would I Do It Again? 21

6. Choosing Your PCP 28

7. Advocate for Yourself. You Deserve the Best! 33

8. Healthcare Roles: Your Hands-on Occupations (This Summary Is Not All-inclusive) 37

9. Hospital Admissions 46

10. Protecting Our Loved Ones: Elder Abuse 53

11. Emergency Plan 56

12. Evolution of Health Insurance:
    A Century of Debate 58

13. Why Do We All Need Some Form of
    Health Insurance? 63

14. Health Insurance Options 65

15. The Health Insurance Debate…Right, or
    Privilege Not Guaranteed? 70

16. PBM: Role of the Pharmacy Benefits
    Managers 72

17. Prescription and Non-prescription
    Medications and Supplements: It Pays to
    Shop! 75

18. The Opioid Epidemic 78

19. Media: The Power of Influence —
    Advertising for New Medications 82

20. Saving Money: Rebates 85

21. Self-pay Patients — How Do They Cope? 87

22. Impact on Losing a Business Due to a
    Catastrophe and No Health Insurance 89

23. The Healthcare Dynasties 92

24. Healthcare for Profit: Awesome Times for Stockholders and CEOs 94

25. My Solution for Providing Healthcare for All in the USA, and I Am Sticking with It. 98

26. Physician Satisfaction...................................... 102

27. The Legal Side of Healthcare 104

28. Healthcare: Yesterday, Today and Tomorrow… 112

29. Final Thoughts on the Financial Side of Healthcare.. 115

About Barb 117

CHAPTER 1
One phone call can change your life and perspective forever

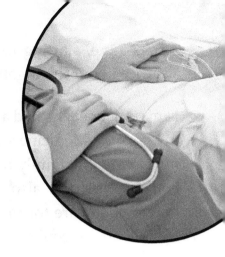

I started writing this book from my perspective as a healthcare provider to empower others in navigating the "business" of healthcare. Ironically and unexpectedly, just as I was finishing the last chapter, I also became a cancer patient...recently diagnosed with amelanotic nodular melanoma. It's an entirely different feeling when you're on the other side as the patient and not the provider of care. The timing of this diagnosis is surreal to me.

My husband Tony and I had finally started closing a couple chapters that were quite stressful and continued to hang over our heads financially for years as a result of my partnership in my old practice. We were starting to explore a few new exciting ideas with joy and anticipation. We were, for a brief time, starting to feel more simplicity and security in our life together.

I am someone who had always put my patients and my job first. Medicine was — and continues to be — my calling. My family has always been important, and my husband also accepted and understood how much I care for my patients. Everything else could wait...or could it?

It's interesting to reflect on these last few months as I was consciously watching a growth on my right arm, and it did not seem that concerning — at least at first. Although it looked ugly, the lesion did not meet the criteria ABCDEs associated with the deadly skin cancer, melanoma, so I thought it was likely benign and something that could wait. So that's what I did.

Meanwhile, I had a little area on my face that wasn't healing, and that was the one I was worried about. My gut was telling me the spot was squamous cell carcinoma (which it was) and that I would be diagnosed, have Mohs surgery, and I was going to be fine.

I continued in observation mode when it came to addressing my right arm lesion. It was symmetrical, round with nice even borders, skin-colored, and still less than the size of a pencil eraser. Excuses kept getting in the way of taking the time to schedule an appointment. I really felt the worst-case scenario was that I would have a biopsy and have a Mohs procedure, and that would be it.

It was early January and we were going through lots of changes in my new job with Premise Health at Insight Enterprises. We rebranded our clinic and we accomplished serious growth in the last few months' time. I was so excited and proud, as the clinic was vibrant and patients were getting the care that they deserved. I had put best practices to use from my twenty years of building practices, and it worked! At the same time, we had major staffing changes and were preparing for the launch of Epic, our new EMR (electronic medical record).

Within the last few weeks of March, the arm lesion grew bigger and uglier. The D and E portions of the ABCDEs now applied. The lesion was growing fast and was bigger than the tip of a pencil eraser.

I had a patient in the office with a similar lesion on his arm, and I referred him to my dermatology group: Skin and Cancer Center of Arizona. After his biopsy, he was diagnosed with nodular basal cell carcinoma. I wondered at that point if perhaps my lesion was also basal cell, as it looked so similar. Even if that were the case, I thought it could wait. I felt well. I was just a little tired, but that was to be expected with longer hours and everything going on at work.

At the same time, I've been charging ahead to complete this book…driven to share my twenty years of knowledge and medical experience to advocate for others so they can feel empowered and have great healthcare experiences. No matter what, I was going to get my book published by early this year. I had procrastinated long enough.

During this time, I also launched my Ask the PA show, Best of Health at PBRX radio. Great people and stories were being showcased. I continued to be so excited and even launched our Dementia Show the day after I had my biopsies.

Today as I continue to advocate for myself, I have to thank my husband Tony who insisted I go to the dermatologist. Tony made the appointment, and there were no openings until May. Four days later I had an appointment after texting my amazing friend and dermatologist PA Beth Lopez, at Tony's insistence. I'm grateful to Beth for her compassion and willingness to see me for an evaluation so quickly. That very appointment may have saved my life.

Let's Talk Melanoma

Less than 2% of the population will get melanoma, and I was diagnosed with a rare form called amelanotic nodular melanoma. This form of melanoma accounts for less than 8% of all melanoma diagnosed. Unfortunately, this type has a different appearance from other types of melanoma. Amelanotic melanomas are missing the pigment typical in most melanomas and can resemble other types of skin cancers such as basal cell or squamous cell carcinoma, or unfortunately may be mistaken for benign moles, warts, or cysts. I beat myself up a bit for being so naïve, as I had diagnosed many melanomas over the years. This was different, but no excuses.

As far as my skin cancer risk, I did get a lot of sunburns/blistering as a child growing up at the Jersey shore. I never really was a sunbather, and I used sunscreens most of the time. I have attempted to keep covered up while out in the sun. We have friends in Mexico where we visit frequently, and they have asked why we were so "white" living in Arizona. Some would tease me about my lack of showing skin to avoid the sun. **Despite that, it still got me.**

My journey so far:

Once diagnosed, I met with my oncologist, Dr. Sujith R. Kalmadi, at Ironwood Cancer and Research Center. He went through my reports and ordered labs and a PET scan. I was also referred to Dr. Mark Runfola at Advanced Surgical Associates. He explained what to expect and told me I had a 1-4 chance of metastasis to my lymph nodes. Just to be sure, along with a wide excision of the cancer, he would remove 2-3 nodes from my axilla (armpit). The next week I had surgery.

My surgery went well, and I was left with a 7-inch long scar on my arm. This will serve as a not-so-gentle reminder of this life-changing moment.

The PET scan has confirmed that at this point the cancer has not spread throughout my body, and this brings me hope. The next step was finding out whether all the cancer has been removed and whether my lymph nodes are negative.

The following week, I had the Mohs surgery with Dr. Joseph Janik at Skin and Cancer Center of AZ, and plastic surgery closure with Dr. Jennifer Boll in Tempe. Those procedures went as expected, and I am healing nicely.

That same day I received a phone call from Dr. Runfola with my results. The good news was they got all the cancer at the original site. The tissue around it looked good and the lymph nodes looked small and healthy, but...two of the three were positive for microscopic metastasis, less than 1mm. I wanted to cry. Now what? In the back of my mind, after a lot of research, I thought to myself, *Even if the doctors tell me I'm OK, I wonder about that one rogue cell that can potentially multiply and wreak more havoc someday.* As I tried to take this in, I found myself thinking, *I am the 1-4 and now I am officially Stage 3A.* We chatted a few more minutes, and after all my data was run through a risk-assessment tool, the result showed that I had around a 30% chance of recurrence of this cancer some-where else, or a new cancer. All I could think was *Now what?*

I called Dr. Kalmadi and had lots of questions. I was not going to wait two weeks to ask. I was in advocate mode for myself. He most graciously saw me and let me know that as a result of this I would qualify for immunotherapy. I had read so many articles and also stories of people's jour-neys. The thought of doing nothing other than three-month screenings, scans in a few months, and waiting, to me was a guarantee I would likely in time be diagnosed with metastatic melanoma, and that was not an acceptable plan. I was in-formed that the FDA approved immunotherapy for those at Stage 3 advanced melanoma. The re-sults of the trials have been very encouraging and so I am excited to have the opportunity to have this therapy.

I was placed on Opdivo (Nivolumab). It specifi-cally helps your immune system attack and kill the cancer cells while protecting your healthy cells. I have had eleven infusions to date, and so far so good. This medicine is also helping people with specific lung cancers and other cancers, with impressive results. This newer therapy is bringing many people hope and longer survival rates. Fingers crossed that it will do the same for me.

I'm beyond grateful for the treatment I've had so far, and I'm confident that close follow-up and these therapies will save my life. I am tough, and I'm a fighter. I also believe there's so much more to be done, and this setback has motivated me even more to try and help others get the best care possible - whether you are a patient, advocate or provider.

I am so grateful for the wonderful care of my Melanoma team: Tony, Beth Lopez PA-C, Dr. Neil Fernandes, Dr. Mark Runfola, Dr. Sujith Kalmadi and their amazing staffs. I really hope you learn a lot from my book and follow my journey, as I truly believe I can be an influencer for change.

As I reflect on my very first Ask the PA video, my topic was the importance of having access to some form of health insurance – whether you're in the United States or elsewhere. Part of this book delves into insurance, and I am experiencing firsthand the importance of having catastrophic health insurance. I'm also a huge proponent of Health

Savings Account (HSA) plans. My HSA plan has a $4,500 deductible and my maximum out of pocket expense is $6,500. In less than one week since my cancer diagnosis, I have blown through that amount and am grateful that my insurance will cover a majority of the rest. If it weren't for health insurance, Tony and I would be in financial ruin.

Here's to you and your *Best of Health*!
I hope you enjoy my book...

CHAPTER 2
Helping You Survive the "Business" of Healthcare: Knowledge Is Power!

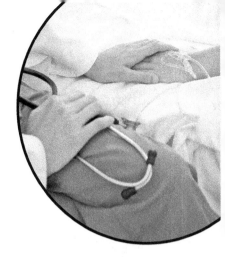

I am a Physician Assistant who has been caring for patients for over 20 years. Family Practice — cradle to grave — is my specialty.

Following the footsteps of three generations of family practice physicians (my father, grandfather, and great-grandfather), this was a natural and genetic calling that I am deeply proud of. Given this, I have a unique perspective, and it's time to share that information. Throughout this book, I also want to give you glimpses of those events from my childhood that influenced my approach to healthcare and shaped who I am today.

As a healthcare provider, teacher, business owner, patient, and advocate for my family and friends throughout the years, I have been painfully aware that there are disconnects with the current state of healthcare in the US and throughout the world. It can be confusing and frankly, very scary.

My goal through this book is to provide information that will empower you to make better healthcare decisions for you and your family. I want to help you navigate through a confusing system, get the right answers, and share ways to save money and time along the way. Helping you prepare for the unexpected is also a major focus here.

I aim to offer thoughts and opinions based on years of my experience and passion. Sharing information for dialogue and discussions may change how you think and approach your health moving forward.

Educate, Empower, and Execute is the ultimate goal.

Here's to your best health!

CHAPTER 3
Following in My Dad's Footsteps

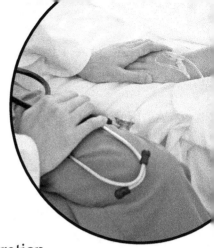

My dad was the third generation of physicians, as my great-grandfather had been a medical missionary in the early 1900s. My grandfather (mom's father) had a practice out of his house in Yonkers, New York. His plan was to have his son-in law go back to New York after medical school and practice with him. That was not my mom's plan, so after residency, my parents landed in a small southeastern Pennsylvania town (Coopersburg) with a population of around 1,800.

My dad recalls the struggles he had setting up his practice on Main Street and having a hard time finding financing. The Coopersburg Bank was also on Main Street, but they did not want to deal with him, so he ended up getting a loan for his start-up from a bank in Quakertown, which was only five miles away. He remained very loyal to them, as they gave him the break he needed so that he could serve his community.

As his business became successful, Dad said that up until the day he left his practice he was approached by the bank on Main Street but he always said no...he was a very loyal man. It's funny, because when my business partner and I opened our practice in 2003, we ran into the same situation. Years later, when our practice showed financial stability, many commercial bankers reached out and wanted to do business - an example of how certain aspects of business do not change.

Best of health!

A glimpse into our not-so-sleepy town...

Our town: Coopersburg, Pennsylvania

Like most quaint towns in the '70s, we had a volunteer fire department and a funeral home. We also had Mack the Mayor, Officer Snyder, and my dad. Whenever anything was going on in our not-so-sleepy town, these three superheroes were usually the first responders before the rest of the volunteers were aware there was a problem.

Mack the Mayor was also the town barber. Cop Snyder was head of the local police department. Dad was one of the two town docs.

My dad's office, the local grocery store, hardware store, hotel, bar and a barbershop were all located along Main Street. Whether the activity was preparing for a local parade, carnival, soapbox races, or other town event, they all worked together to benefit the rest of us. Kids felt safe, and we were all protected.

My parents slowly built their family practice with Mom as the bookkeeper, and other than a part-time nurse, my dad had no other employees. They remained very discreet about anything related to the families they served. Patient care and confidentiality were the priorities. We even went to church in another town and they did their best to keep our lives as a family separate.

In those days HIPAA did not exist, and health insurance was still evolving. People without insurance were charged a fair price or bartered for services rendered. In some ways, it was so much simpler.

Oh, how things have changed.

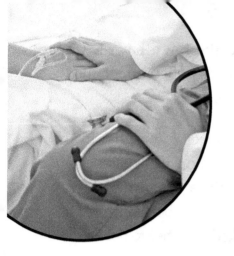

CHAPTER 4

*Why I Love Being
a Primary Care
Provider (PCP)*

Scenario:

Mary was seen in the ER and also cardiology for heart palpitations. She was cleared by both specialties after evaluation. She referred herself to me because she did not feel well and proceeded to tell me her symptoms such as anxiety, weight loss, loose stools, and her heart would race at times. Throughout her course of care, one would hope that someone had checked her thyroid. Sadly, no one had.

After her appointment, I ordered a thyroid panel and also thyroid antibodies. Upon review of her lab results, I diagnosed Mary with hyperthyroidism. We discussed that this could be concerning, so she agreed to a thyroid ultrasound as well as some additional studies. Her final diagnosis after a thyroid biopsy was thyroid cancer. Following appropriate treatment, Mary has been cured!

I love being a primary care provider, as I get to care for people from cradle to grave. I specialize in preventive medicine and also pride myself on being a good diagnostician. Back in the day when my father and those before him practiced medicine, there were not so many specialists out there to work with. Today, we have so many levels of specialty it is mind-boggling.

As the PCP, not only am I able to help you with a lot of your medical problems; it is also my role to advise on the correct specialist to see. Many times over the years, I have had referrals from specialists because the patient had no PCP. If these people had seen me first, they potentially could have saved money and in some instances avoided the specialists altogether.

This is why I love my job!

A glimpse into our not-so-sleepy town…

Medicine as seen through a child's eyes

Imagine the early '70s, living in a home where Dad's office was on the first floor and my bedroom was right above the front door. There was only one other local doctor, and between the two of them, they cared for a few thousand patients in our town and also other nearby communities. Our residence on Main Street was not only the location of my dad's practice, but it was our family home. Friends and relatives gathered for social occasions, and I would have sleepovers with my friends.

Imagine back then being a kid and hearing the doorbell ring in the middle of the night. Dad would get up to greet whoever was at the front door, and I remember hearing the familiar phrase, "Hold on one second. I'll go open up the office."

My father not only saw patients from cradle to grave, he also delivered many babies along the way. Quite a few holidays went by with Dad nowhere to be found because he was at the hospital delivering another baby. We would postpone celebrating Christmas until he arrived home, with the exception of Mom letting us open one gift in the morning. The rest would wait to be opened until Dad came home. He sometimes had to leave to make a last-minute emergency house call, and we would wait for Dad before leaving for whatever occasion as a family. Mom was amazing in the way she supported him and us no matter what happened. No day was ever the same. Their norm for us was adapting to the needs of the patients and Dad's practice.

His practice consisted of a part-time nurse and my mom, his bookkeeper. He also made house calls daily and spent hours following up on any of his patients admitted to the hospital. My father charged nine dollars for an office visit and never demanded payment the day of service. My mom's bookkeeping system was a file with cardboard charts. Back then if someone did not have cash, Dad also accepted chickens, fish, and food and even bartered a lot for services around the house.

From the beginning my parents worked very hard, but my mom made sure that we all, as a family, played hard too. We were involved in school activities. For me it was horses, golf, and music. We took routine vacations and enjoyed time at the shore.

A tradition I loved took place on Presidents Day weekend. We drove to Atlantic City and stayed at a hotel on the boardwalk. We would walk the boards in our winter coats, swim in the heated pool, and have dinner at the same restaurant year after year, where we enjoyed Italian food and the best cheesecake ever. Traditions like that kept us grounded as a family.

CHAPTER 5
Why a Physician Assistant (PA)? Would I Do It Again?

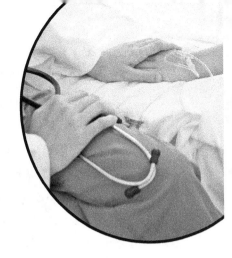

I knew at an early age that I would ultimately end up in family medicine. I was in a health science pre-med class in sixth grade and also loved anatomy. We had an amazing science teacher. A group of us ended up in an advanced science elective. We got to dissect frogs and other small animals. I also loved golf and my music. Since fourth grade, I had studied privately and was becoming more accomplished. As a result, I had opportunities to study with great musicians and ultimately go to college on a music performance scholarship. I love music, and I know that discipline and creativity helped me become a much more confident person. I transitioned to medicine in my early thirties, after a successful teaching career as a musician.

Once I started in my practice as a PA, I had lofty goals of setting up a private practice, teaching, and leadership. The PA profession was still in its infancy and many did not understand our training and our capability as providers. We were still on the frontier as we all forged ahead in the profession to gain understanding and acceptance. Back then, I began to realize that being a physician would have likely been a better fit, as I was met with obstacles along the way as a PA. I can remember being on call for the County in 1999 and an emergency doctor refusing to talk to me and only wanting to converse with a "real provider."

Fortunately, I was able to accomplish many of my goals, but only with help from my family, friends, and some amazing PAs and physicians who believed in me. I will never forget the ongoing support from our staff and my patients as well. Today, several years later, I am often asked if I would make the career change to medicine again. The answer is yes!

What I Learned:

Given the current state of the "business side" of medicine, and if I had been given the gift of foresight, I likely would have become a Medical Doctor (MD) or a Doctor of Osteopathic Medicine (DO). As a physician, I would have had more leverage with career decisions. As a PA starting out, there were not many opportunities for advancement. The profession was still young, and many people in and out of healthcare struggled with the PA's place in medicine. We have come a long way since 1997.

As an aspiring owner of a family practice, in the early 2000s I found my opportunity, although I thought it would be a lot easier than it turned out. As the PA and head of Operations, I had a great partner and we believed we could make a difference...and we did. Our team worked extremely hard, and our patients received great care but with a huge sacrifice on our end. It took much longer to stabilize financially than anyone could have imagined. Many aspects, including the economy, played a factor. Each step was a challenge, but looking back on it, I really grew and learned many lessons along the way.

Opening a medical practice taught me how to prioritize business decisions more thoughtfully by analyzing the critical essentials to opening the door versus what could wait. I have a huge appreciation for that now! For me personally, I learned a lot from the school of hard knocks and frankly from the lack of a solid business plan. These days, before I would ever entertain the idea of another practice, I would get a MBA or consider bringing in a strong business manager.

I hope that my experience and advice can help you, whether you are just curious about the business side of medicine or you are an aspiring healthcare professional. Don't we all want to achieve our dreams? We spend more time at our careers than we do at home, and it had better be a good fit!

A glimpse into our not-so-sleepy town…

The Explosion

I remember vividly that day in fifth grade. I was at school in our hometown and we had just gotten into the cafeteria for lunch. Out of nowhere, we heard a very loud boom. The pots and pans hanging from the ceiling in the kitchen were banging together and falling. Shortly after that, a second boom hit. The teachers and staff quickly assembled all of us on the playground in our respective classes. Behind us, about a block away, was a dark plume of thick, scary smoke. There was confusion as to what had just happened. Teachers were trying to comfort us, but we knew they were worried too. I just wanted to go home.

At that time before cell phones, there was no way to notify parents about an early release from school, but we were sent home for our safety. A group of us were walking north toward my house on Main Street and the burning apartment building was in the opposite direction. As we looked down the street we saw fragments of cassette tapes, eight tracks, and toys along the sidewalk and in the front yards of our neighbors' homes.

As I arrived at the front door of my house, I said goodbye to my friends. I walked up the steps onto our porch, and I remember looking through the window as I slowly opened the door. People were gathered in our living room. I could smell coffee and also noticed some desserts that Mom was preparing in the kitchen for our visitors. When Mom and I finally saw each other, she gave me a big hug and held me for a few seconds.

Strangers filled every corner of our home. Mom quietly explained that they were family members of people involved in the gas explosion, which she said happened at the apartment building across from Mack's barbershop.

My father was down with Mack and the volunteer fire department helping to rescue and recover people trapped in the rubble. I sat back and watched the events of that afternoon unfold as people were desperately waiting for information about their loved ones. People were identifying jewelry and other small personal items that were brought to our home. It was a sad day for all of us as we learned the fate of neighbors' loved ones. Back then, there were no paid EMS, firefighters, or paramedics. Everybody was a volunteer.

Later it was determined that the gas explosion had been set off by a blow torch used to repair the sewer line. An electrician using the blow torch had been a family friend and my dad's patient. He along with five others passed away that horrific day.

For a few days we had to go to a different school until ours was declared safe, and for a few nights after the explosion I was on edge because I wasn't sure if it was going to happen again. I could still smell the rubble and worried that our house would be next. Finally, I would fall asleep. I knew my parents were close by, and that brought comfort, knowing we were all together.

I learned a lot from watching my parents. My father was a hero and my mom a gracious hostess. Our home was a place of comfort and calm. I reflect on this time of my life now and I could not be prouder of them.

That's what medicine and healthcare was all about in those days!

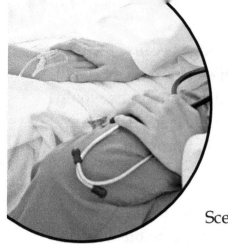

CHAPTER 6
Choosing Your PCP

Scenario:

John came in with his wife for his first appointment. Their body language told me that they were not eager to be there. They proceeded to tell me that he had become more emotionally erratic and that he had been to two other providers thus far seeking answers. He had no history of emotional problems with himself or his family.

He was happy overall but indicated moments of crying for no reason. No workup had been done prior to his appointment that day; he was diagnosed with depression, given an anti-depressant (SSRI), and also told he was going through a nervous breakdown. He assured me he was not depressed and that he had no reason for a breakdown. He feared that he might lose his job over his sudden outbursts. We had a long chat and after diving into these concerns, I ordered labs and imaging. We also slowly weaned him off the SSRI.

When John's studies came back, he was diagnosed with a brain tumor! Luckily it was benign, and today he is cured. His erratic behavior stopped after the surgery and he is back to being the John his wife loves.

Recommendation:

As a Primary Care Provider (PCP) and also a patient myself, I believe that the most important component for a meaningful healthcare experience is connecting with someone who listens and cares.

Researching your potential PCP is important, and I feel strongly that word of mouth is the key. To be able to obtain the best of health requires being honest and expressing your concerns. Let your provider hear you, and insist that he or she has the whole story.

Rome was not built in a day; obtaining the best care possible takes time. Invest the time in yourself! Be patient!

Consider your first appointment as a consultation and accept that many times health concerns have accumulated over time, so it takes time to connect and put the entire story together. As long as you are moving forward, you are on your way! If you feel rushed and unheard, then find another PCP.

It is also important as a medical provider to take the time to listen, step back, and engage. It is so worth it and so rewarding!

A glimpse into our not-so-sleepy town…

The Arson

It was never boring in Coopersburg. Everybody knew each other. My father was also the team doctor for the local high school. My oldest brother, who today is an accomplished disc jockey/program director for a radio station in central Pennsylvania, was the announcer for our hometown Little League.

It was summer, and we were in the middle of baseball season. One night, our town's Little League stadium burned to the ground. There was nothing left of the building that supported the dugouts, refreshments, and my brother's announcing booth.

As you can imagine, our family was devastated. This is where we went for many baseball games and also to hear my brother announce. It was gone! The investigation pointed to arson. But who?

A few days later, Dad was in his office with patients and Mom was in the kitchen when a family friend knocked on the back door of our house. He walked into the kitchen very calmly and said, "I need to talk to Doc now." Mom invited him to sit down. Several minutes later my dad came out of his office and greeted our friend and asked me to leave the room, so I headed out back to play. I was used to that routine when privacy was requested, and I knew not to come back in the home until they opened the door.

The person we all knew and cared for as a friend and mentor for my brother admitted to my parents that he burned down the Little League stadium. He proceeded to explain why, although it really didn't matter, considering what was done was done. A few minutes later our town officer, Cop Snyder, arrived, and our friend was placed in cuffs and we never saw him again. This had a lasting effect on many people, including my family.

My parents knew many of the teachers, coaches, business people, and families as patients and friends. I can only imagine how difficult it was keeping everyone's secrets to themselves. That's exactly what they did.

CHAPTER 7
Advocate for Yourself. You Deserve the Best!

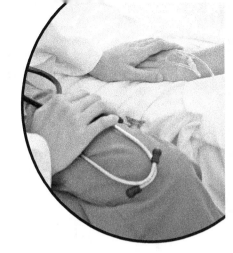

What would you do?

Scenario:

Tommy, a veteran who served in Vietnam, gets his healthcare through a well-known government agency that starts with a V. He is in his sixties and is very active. He was recently diagnosed with prostate cancer, but to this point they have not released the pathology and staging results to him. He is told he may likely live ten years with it and is given a pamphlet called "Living with Prostate Cancer."

As practitioners, many are taught to base their clinical decision-making on evidence-based medicine (EBM). EBM treatment options are recommended based on studies and statistics rather than any patient input. This is clearly what happened here.

Tommy insisted that his pathology results be released to him. He reached out to a local private urologist and learned about his options. He was able to get treatment and is now cured.

Thoughts:

I have always felt strongly that providers should focus on and respect patient expectations. Patients' wishes must be taken into consideration during the clinical decision-making process. After all, whose life is it?

As a provider, over the years I have encouraged my patients to get second opinions. If you have a provider who is hesitant to refer you to another provider, then go shopping for a new provider.

A glimpse into our not-so-sleepy town…

The Murder

Our town was located along Route 309 between Allentown and Quakertown and was rich in tradition. Several generations of families had their roots there with many births, weddings, funerals, annual picnics, parades, and social gatherings. My favorite was the annual carnival, which everyone looked forward to!

We also had heartbreak. Unfortunately, given my dad's job, my parents knew everyone in town—not by choice but by profession. This really hit home in 1973.

A very special young man my parents had known years ago as a Boy Scout in their troop later went to high school with my brothers and had a part-time job at a gas station south of town on Route 309. One day in 1973, everything changed when he was kidnapped and murdered by one of our neighbors after a robbery at that gas station went terribly wrong. He was sixteen years old.

Not everyone can stay neutral when tragedy strikes, but my parents did. Over the years, they cared not only for the family of the murdered young man, but also for the family of the murderer. Mom had personal relationships with both of these mothers, one being a neighbor and one a fellow troop mom. Well, you can guess Dad's relationship in trying to heal two families in a small town destroyed by grief and confusion. Everyone went on in our community, but things were never quite the same.

Medicine in the late '60s, '70s, and early '80s as I experienced it was quite a different profession from what it is today. It was personal, and it was your life. Memories as a child and young adult have greatly influenced who I am today.

CHAPTER 8
Healthcare Roles: Your Hands-on Occupations (This Summary Is Not All-inclusive)

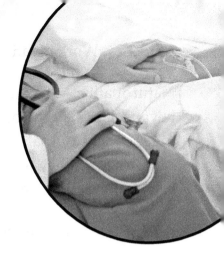

There is so much confusion concerning many of the "hands-on" medical players. All these folks can play a role in both the inpatient and outpatient environments. This is not complete but a great start in understanding why healthcare will never lack for jobs, especially as our population continues to grow. Let me emphasize that in addition to the roles listed below, there are many more opportunities in administrative and support roles in the healthcare experience.

Physicians

Medical Doctor (MD)/Doctor of Osteopathic Medicine (DO) – Attend medical school and residency. Work inpatient/outpatient and research.

Naturopaths - Advanced training for four years beyond their bachelor's degree. They can have independent outpatient practices. Although they can prescribe, they focus on alternative treatments such as herbal, vitamin, and hormone therapy.

Advanced Care Providers

Physician Assistants (PAs) – Attend PA school after undergraduate education with most schools at the master's degree level. Training, as with physicians, is based on the medical model. PAs work collaboratively with physicians in primary care and many specialty settings. The profession, unlike the Nurse Practitioner, requires a supervising agreement with a physician.

Nurse Practitioners (NPs) – Attend NP school after undergraduate education with minimally a master's degree. They are trained based on the nursing model. In seven states, they can set up practices and work independently without any physician supervision or collaboration.

Behavioral Health

Psychiatrists – MDs/DOs who have additional training (residency) in psychiatry and/or mental health.

Clinical Psychologists – Advanced training at usually the doctorate level. Many have their own practices, but also many focus on behavioral research and analytics. They can't write prescriptions.

Counselors – Advanced training at the master's level. Can practice independently in some states.

Ancillary Providers

Physical Therapists (PTs) – Work with issues "below the waist"; they can be found in both inpatient and outpatient settings. They assess strength and ability to ambulate (walk). They specialize in rehabilitation after injuries or surgeries on the knees, hips, legs, or feet. They can also work with fitting prosthetics.

Occupational Therapists (OTs) - Help patients with anything "above the waist"; they are hand therapists and also help with improving activities of daily living (ADL) in inpatient and outpatient settings. They help people relearn to cook, shave, bathe, and dress.

Speech Therapists – Evaluate and treat patients with speech as well as issues with swallowing in both inpatient and outpatient settings.

Respiratory Therapists – Work in primarily inpatient settings, but also provide home health and testing on pulmonary issues such as asthma or COPD.

Registered Dietitians – Evaluate and make recommendations concerning meals and dietary needs upon assessment. They also have outpatient opportunities in their own practices and work with cancer centers and other hospital specialties providing nutrition advice and counseling.

Nursing Staff

Nurses – Have minimally an associate's degree but many go on to obtain bachelor's degrees in nursing. They are, in my opinion, the hospital heroes. They follow through with provider orders and perform nursing assessments and lead their teams. They have amazing opportunities for work in both inpatient and outpatient settings.

Nursing Assistants – Work in the hospital setting, nursing homes and home health, and in many outpatient settings. Assist the nursing staff with bathing, meds, and patient care and comfort as designated.

Medical Assistants – Work in outpatient clinics, primarily doing tasks such as rooming, vitals, EKGs, labs, and other patient care as designated by their provider.

Phlebotomists – Work primarily drawing blood and performing lab tasks in both inpatient and outpatient settings in medical offices, hospitals, and labs.

Radiology Technicians (Radiographers) – Perform imaging in both inpatient and outpatient environments. They have a minimum of an associate's degree and advanced certifications are required for ultrasound, CT, MRI.

Paramedics and Technicians – Can be found working in hospitals (ER) and work in the field as the first line.

I want to share this information to give you an idea of some of the many possible healthcare career options. Also, if you or a loved one is hospital-ized, it is not uncommon to be seen by many of the above listed professions and it can be confusing to understand their individual roles in your care.

In my dad's three-day hospitalization in recent years for complications of influenza and electro-lyte imbalance, he had been evaluated and cared for by the following:

MD (hospitalist), NP, psychiatrist, PT, OT, speech therapist, respiratory therapist, registered dieti-tian, nurses, a nursing assistant, phlebotomists, ra-diology techs, and he was brought to the ER by the paramedics.

No wonder he complained about never getting any rest!

A glimpse into our not-so-sleepy town…

The Decision for Change

I was in sixth grade, and at that point my dad's practice was huge. He had been in practice for about twenty years. He continued to work hard and play hard, but he had a sense that a change needed to happen - but what? My oldest brother was in college and my middle brother was in tenth grade. I was twelve years old and in middle school.

Dad seemed tired and a bit withdrawn. The everyday pace was getting to him physically and emotionally. Mom also felt a sense of restlessness and uneasiness, as she was also trying to care for my grandparents. This required her to travel back and forth to New York. Balancing her responsibilities raising us and caring for her parents was taking a toll.

I recall Dad discussing that a few physicians he knew were getting ill and one friend had a heart attack. The practice became more and more demanding on him as he tried to juggle his workload with family obligations. He was in his early fifties and tired. Dad considered rejoining the military as he had served in the Navy during WWII. He also contemplated moving us to the Jersey shore to practice with a friend from medical school.

Right before the decision to move, I remember fondly spending a summer at the shore while Dad worked urgent care there. He was testing the waters for a move to the shore. It was a great time for me spending six weeks with him. I learned to sail a sunfish that summer. I worked at the marina in exchange for lessons. After work, Dad would go fishing, or we would just hang out together. Mom and my brother would visit often, as she was juggling her responsibilities with her parents. My oldest brother was working at a local radio station at the shore for the summer.

My parents' priorities were to provide a stable education and positive environment for us. Given this, the military option of Dad re-enlisting in the Navy as an officer was not a fit, since we would not have stability as a family. Dad also realized that working with a new partner at the Jersey shore would be essentially starting a new practice with similar stressors all over again. He also felt that we would not have a good education, after researching the public schools there.

My dad and mom announced the closing of his practice for a move to Indiana, PA where he would practice as a physician on campus at Indiana University of Pennsylvania (IUP). I knew deep down that this would be something new and a welcome opportunity for all of us. However, moving away from my friends and activities was really difficult for me as a teenager in eighth grade. Once we moved, I was resentful at first and not so nice. New school and trying to fit in had their challenges. It just took time.

Leaving our small town meant my parents could have a personal life and be themselves for the first time without the daily pressures. They would have set schedules and be more involved with us. Dad immediately involved himself in the campus and some organizations such as the Lions Club. We went to church in the same town, and Mom and Dad were quickly developing strong, lasting friendships.

A fun side note: A doctor from the next town over from Coopersburg bought Dad's practice, and a dentist bought our house. He renovated the home office for his dental practice. A year later, a small three-doctor practice moved into town to continue to care for the families and friends in Coopersburg and the Lehigh Valley.

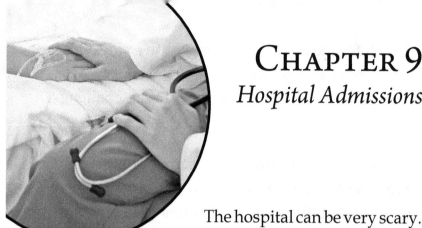

CHAPTER 9
Hospital Admissions

The hospital can be very scary. If your loved one is admitted to the hospital, it's critical that you keep your eye on what's going on. Never hesitate to ask a question. It's important that you make sure they know your loved one's history, medications, allergies, primary care provider, and specialists. Even as Electronic Medical Records (EMRs) are getting more connected, we still have a long way to go in tracking our own personal information; in the meantime, there are some great apps available to keep track of your medical history and meds. If you are not computer savvy, bring in the medications to your provider or take photos of the bottles.

It's also important that you share with the providers and nurses exactly what the patient's baseline was before being admitted to the hospital. This is critical for the elderly; otherwise they will be dismissed. Show photos or whatever it takes to create a connection with the inpatient team.

Years ago, your doctor would be your hospitalist, but these days it's pretty rare. The hospitalist is an internist in charge of the care of your loved one while in the hospital and is responsible for orchestrating specialty referrals, tests, and care throughout the hospital stay and making sure the patient has a smooth transition out.

I truly believe the nursing staff is the team that makes or breaks the hospitalization. It's critical that you let them know what the patient is used to as far as activities of daily living. Don't make assumptions. For example, my father is easy going but he likes to be clean, so all he ever wants is a shower, his hair combed, and to make sure his teeth are brushed every day. Unfortunately, when he was admitted, he went a day or two without those basic needs being addressed. For some people, missing a shower may not be a big deal, but for my father, it was.

Never assume that the patient is unaware of what's going on around him or her. My father, who is over ninety, felt in his last hospitalization that his hospitalist dismissed him. Dad was very aware, and he was taken aback when his doctor talked *about* him, but not *to* him. He said that he was not even examined. As a retired doctor, he was not at all satisfied with this experience. As a doctor, who in the day, charged $9 for a visit, he was also a bit shocked when the hospitalist was paid $200 for, in my father's opinion, five minutes tops.

Hospital Discharge

If everything goes smoothly in the hospital, the next step is making sure the transitional piece is in place. This can be even more frustrating. In my father's situation, would he go to rehabilitation or back home? With his flu diagnosis, even though he was very weak, he was sent home.

Finding Home Health

You are given a list of agencies, or if you are lucky, at discharge this is arranged. For example, if you need a nurse assessment along with PT and OT, the agency is selected, and you are given a phone number and the agency gets your number. By some miracle this follow-up piece gets coordinated.

Caregivers

If you need additional caregivers to help at home, many times you are given a list and the hunt is on. In our case we needed someone for morning help for a few days. We called multiple agencies and heard every excuse. "The location is too far." "We don't help people with the flu." "We are short staffed." "We can't get anyone out to do an assessment for a few days." We ended up helping Dad ourselves.

It would be great to have a streamlined process to be able to find the correct match. Many times, you just have to take your chances and hope for the best.

Medications

Never assume anything, so double check medications upon discharge. Also, make sure you were given all the correct prescriptions before you leave. Double check names and the doses, and if you have any questions…ASK.

Scenario:

This happened in our family at a rehabilitation facility. My dad was transferred to a facility, and I reviewed the medications the nurse was going to give him. We were all tired, and Dad was not out of the woods. He was not at all mentally or physically the man I know and love. One of the medications on his discharge paperwork that was to be given to him that evening at the rehab facility was a medication that contributed to his hospital admission in the first place.

I told the nurse not to give that drug to my dad. She refused. You can only imagine, as a healthcare provider, how I felt. It was a Sunday and his new doctor would not be available until the morning. The nurse could not reach him or maybe she did not want to. It was very disturbing to me. I told her simply not to give the med, as I am his advocate and she could feel free to record on his chart: "against medical advice". I did not care. He was not going to get it and if he did, who knows what could have happened. Many people die annually due to medication errors.

Living Wills

Everyone really needs to consider this, and a living will can be made at no charge. It is our nature to want to speak and make decisions for ourselves. Why is this different? This is another subject many just do not think of or want to talk about. My gut feeling is that many of us believe it will never be needed, so why bother? This can affect any of us at any time and at any age.

Scenario:

Your seventy-year-old grandmother has a stroke and ends up in the emergency room. She told you previously that she never wants CPR to revive her and does not want to be intubated. With no living will documenting her wishes, the heroic providers decide to intubate and do whatever it takes to keep her alive. They also end up placing a feeding tube. After all this, it is determined that there is no hope and she is in an indefinite coma. Her EEG shows no brain activity. Now the pain begins as to what to do to honor her wishes.

Solution:

Especially with the elderly, a living will is critical. Each state has some twists so make sure you are covered legally and it is updated.

By having each person's wishes known, we can avoid so much pain and suffering. People get their wishes honored and the family has peace of mind with direction to do what's right with no drama and no court orders.

Many online sources are available to complete these forms. There are also cost-effective paralegal services, as well as estate planners. You do not need to hire a fancy expensive law firm. Just do your homework!

Once the forms are completed and notarized, please share that information with any designated family member(s).

Your primary care provider can also provide and store a copy for you and get it to the hospital quickly when requested.

Chapter 10
*Protecting Our
Loved Ones:
Elder Abuse*

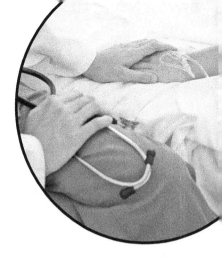

Elder abuse is a general term used to describe harmful acts toward an elderly adult. This can be physical abuse, sexual abuse, emotional or psychological abuse, financial exploitation, and neglect, including self-neglect.

Unfortunately, this is rampant, and it seems to get minimal attention until after someone is a victim. As we age it is natural to experience memory issues and become more trusting and lonely. This is a perfect scenario for predators to prey on the vulnerable among us.

Certain life events can make the elderly more vulnerable, such as an illness or death of a loved one. Many abusers can research someone's life through hard print or social media. It's scary to think how easy it is for these individuals to set up their victims to believe a relationship exists or existed in the past by engaging them in topics such as previous homes, neighbors, or relationships. When one is alone, it is unfortunate, but many fall into the trap out of excitement or at times fear of loneliness. Never be afraid to question your loved one if something does not fit.

As a caregiver and family member who has elderly parents, it is a balancing act for me to encourage independence and not be too hovering, while also making sure they are safe from predators.

We experienced these challenges in our family numerous times with the death of my father-in-law, as well as threatening phone scams aimed at my parents. To avoid future phone scams, we now pay for a phone line that prohibits unsolicited calls. That has helped a lot, and my parents are happier not dealing with all the unnecessary calls.

We also learned that when a loved one has new acquaintances and doesn't want to at least introduce these new acquaintances to family, have your guard up. That is not healthy, and this secretive relationship can result in long-lasting abuse and fraud.

Elder abuse can happen anywhere and at any time. Be vigilant. Never make assumptions. Any time there is a transition, elders are more vulnerable. It can be as simple as a new home, church, senior center, or medical facility. Watch for signs and changes in behavior. Abuse is all too common, so be observant.

If something seems wrong and does not add up, it likely is.

Best of health!

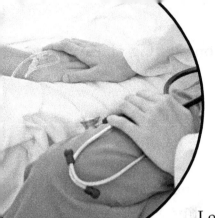

CHAPTER 11
Emergency Plan

Let's face it. No one wants to think this can happen to themselves or their family member, but then the unthinkable happens:

- ✓ Your child is ill
- ✓ Accident happens
- ✓ Parent or loved one is having an emergency

Are you ready? Prepare now!

Checklist

1. Insurance information: health and any supplemental
2. Closest and best in-network hospital or urgent care
3. Primary Health Care Provider contact information

4. Specialist names and contact information

5. Health history

6. Medication list

7. Allergies

8. Living will / advance directives

Our goal is to be proactive rather than reactive. This can avoid medical mistakes and ensure you or your family member gets the best care possible.

Let's get that list ready and store it in a place with easy access.

Best of health!

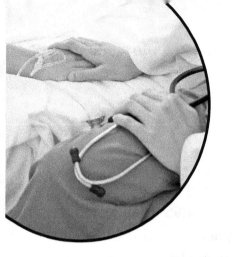

CHAPTER 12
*Evolution of
Health Insurance:
A Century of Debate*

A brief tour:

1900: The start of the revolution of organized medicine. The American Medical Association gained a lot of steam as an organization. Our government had no interest and saw no value in the concept of health insurance. However, European countries did not agree.

1912: Teddy Roosevelt and the Progressive party campaigned for "social insurance." This included health insurance. The American Association of Labor Legislation started promoting the idea of mandatory health insurance. All of this was put on hold when we entered World War I.

1929: The first model for health insurance was introduced when Baylor Hospital initiated a deal with a local teachers' union for prepaid insurance for hospitalizations. This was the beginning of Blue Cross Blue Shield.

1930s: The Great Depression hit, and this was when Franklin Delano Roosevelt (FDR) was able to pass the Social Security Act to protect the elderly. The medical portion (national health insurance), however, was not passed since the American Medical Association opposed it, as they believed it hindered the freedom of doctors to practice and that would affect the patient-provider relationship. They felt there would be too much government control.

1944: FDR introduced the Economic Bill of Rights that emphasized the "right" to medical care. During World War II, businesses started offering health benefits, and this was the beginning of employer-based health insurance.

1945: Harry Truman proposed mandatory coverage, doubling the healthcare workforce. With influence from the AMA as a form of socialized medicine it went nowhere!

1965: Lyndon Baines Johnson (LBJ) signed Medicare and Medicaid into law.

1970s: President Nixon introduced the concept of HMOs to try to reduce costs. These are pre-paid managed care and cheaper options, but with more limitations. Originally, they were non-profit organizations, but once there were for-profit alternatives, patients experienced more and more denials of care. Healthcare became more inefficient, and providers started to see increased workloads.

1980s: Corporations took control. They entered not only the insurance markets but other areas associated with healthcare. In the 1980s we also saw an increase in the number of non-insured to 31 million, or 13 percent of the population.

2006: Massachusetts introduced healthcare reform, sharing the responsibility for health insurance among government, employers, and individuals. Non-insured numbers decreased over 50 percent in the first two years.

2010: The Affordable Care Act (ACA) also known as "Obamacare." The goal was to provide affordable healthcare for all by providing tax credits to businesses and individuals. The hope was to streamline care and bring down costs, help small businesses offer insurance, and enable the self-employed to obtain affordable care. One of the biggest strengths of the ACA was that insurance companies could not decline benefits to those with pre-existing conditions. One of the biggest drawbacks was that, to be successful, it needed everyone to participate and a small penalty was levied for anyone who did not do so. Many elected to pay the penalty instead since the premiums were still too costly.

Insurance companies also were able to opt out, so as of 2017, many states have only one plan to purchase, resulting in premiums skyrocketing.

Did you know also that the ACA bill as voted on was over 2,000 pages? I doubt anyone read it. I truly believe the intent was good, but there were too many loopholes, and we are seeing now the result with rising premiums and less choice. We still have over 27 million Americans, which is about 9%, without health insurance. In 2013 it was significantly higher, hovering around 44 million.

2018: We still struggle with many of the same issues. The ACA is still in place, but for how long, and what will be next? We do know that the US spends more on healthcare than any other country, at over $3 trillion a year. This is hovering around $9,000+ per person.

CHAPTER 13

*Why Do We All
Need Some Form of
Health Insurance?*

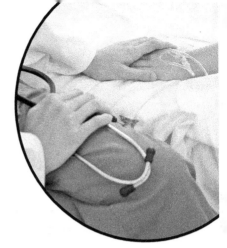

Scenario:

You have no insurance and you end up in the emergency room, diagnosed with appendicitis. Emergency surgery is performed, you stay overnight, and you are sent home to recover.

Your EOB (Explanation of Benefits) arrives and you are stunned as the "usual and customary" rate for your hospital course is $45,000.

The insurance "discounted rate" for the same service would have been $7,800. Yes, the difference can be that inflated, and this is what causes financial devastation overnight.

Solution:

Everyone should consider getting at least a catastrophic policy so you get the "discount." That's defined as the rate each facility and provider negotiates with a particular insurer.

With no insurance, you are billed a "usual and customary" rate and that is super inflated. Not many can afford that.

Research online, and if you are one of those unfortunate people who can't get insurance through an employer or family member, seek out insurance brokers.

Consider trying to obtain the most cost-effective insurance with the highest deductible you can afford. Stick with the more well-known insurers so that you have choices with facilities. Get shopping!

Best of health!

CHAPTER 14
Health Insurance Options

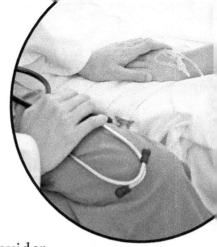

The PPO (Preferred Provider Organization):

For many this is preferred, because the patients have more control over who they ultimately see as their providers of care. It is more expensive but does not require a referral from a primary care provider to consult a specialist.

As long as the facility and provider are in the network, you can be seen. Research your providers, as not all PPOs are equal, and there are restrictions.

The costs associated with PPOs are usually a bit more out of pocket. The deductibles can vary significantly. Once the deductible is met, it's not over. With many plans you, the insured, will still be responsible for a small percentage of your care, usually 10-20% after your deductible is met. You can usually seek care "out of network," but it's going to cost you!

Providers in this PPO model charge, for the most part, fee for service, and they get paid for services rendered. These days, there can be levels of reimbursements based on quality matrices as well.

Also research your prescription benefit, as levels of coverage can vary and some medications can be very expensive. Don't trust the great news that your insurance covers a medication because if it is at a higher tier, your copay can be very significant.

Do your homework!

What's an HMO?

The HMO (Health Maintenance Organization) was developed in the 1970s. It is an alternative form of health insurance where you usually pay cheaper premiums. You are limited to seeing providers in that particular network, including being assigned a PCP (primary care provider). You must go through that provider for all referrals. Many times, the network of providers and facilities is smaller and more limited.

The goal of the HMO is to save money and also keep costs down. In this model, providers get paid a small fee monthly, whether the patient is seen or not. That is referred to as capitation. It sounds great that payment is a fraction of what a provider is paid in the fee-for-service model. However, if providers have a huge panel of HMO patients, it takes away from accessibility. During illness season, good luck getting an appointment.

This model is decent and more cost-effective for the healthy, uncomplicated patient. I do not recommend considering an HMO if you require more complex care and have a circle of providers. Likely, many providers will not take the insurance.

I personally have never liked the model, as it has limitations and short-changes the patient. As a provider who owned my own practice, I felt that the HMO hindered the patient experience and easy access my patients deserve!

The EPO: Exclusive Provider Organization

Just as it sounds, you are required to stay within an exclusive network of providers; otherwise, you are likely not covered if you go out of this network.

Be careful if you have to go out of network for care (especially if you travel). You could get stuck with an unexpected bill.

The High Deductible Health Plan (HDHP) and the HSA Health Savings Accounts

This alternative is a bit more cost-effective for the employer and also for those who are self-employed and have to get insurance on their own! It has really gained in popularity over the last few years.

Yes, it is a higher deductible but this is the only alternative where you can save and accumulate any money that is not used year after year, and the money is pretax. Think of it as another IRA. Once you accumulate a sum— usually greater than $1,600 –you can invest it into electronically traded funds (ETFs).

Many employers will also contribute to this account on your behalf. If you choose this alternative, you can invest it!

Also, you are in a way insuring yourself. Huge win for you if you are healthy.

It's a gift, and people really need to consider researching it!

Many fear not having enough money for health-care costs in retirement, and this is a real solution. Ask your accountants or financial advisors. I know what they will say: Go for it!

Best of health!

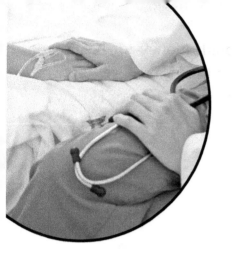

CHAPTER 15
The Health Insurance Debate... Right, or Privilege Not Guaranteed?

Whether we want to admit it, we live in a country where healthcare is deemed a privilege, not a right. It's mind-blowing to me that millions of Americans have no health insurance and, unfortunately, the numbers continue to get bigger. Many families wait to get care until they're in crisis mode and often will seek care outside the country once they get desperate enough. When a working-class family with no health insurance has a crisis, sadly they can even find themselves giving up everything, including their jobs, to get on government assistance.

The United States of America is one of the richest countries in the world and spends more on healthcare per person than essentially every other country. We should look at why it costs so much, and we need to consider other options. Healthcare should never be about the haves and the have-nots. It's providing a service that's imperative to each of us. It's quite obvious that the system is not working.

Over the years I've heard the same story over and over: hard-working family with a small business not being able to afford insurance and going bankrupt after an emergency.

I'm hoping to provide some insight and knowledge throughout this book so that you can make better healthcare decisions. It is my hope that someday every citizen in this country has at least catastrophic coverage for the big stuff. Time will tell.

Best of health!

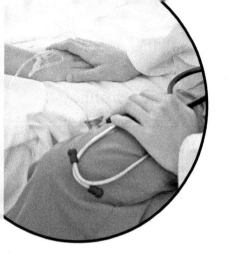

CHAPTER 16
PBM: Role of the Pharmacy Benefits Managers

PBMs are the "middle" people for negotiating down the costs of medications and vaccines. The initial intent was to ensure that large companies, Medicare, and the federal government would get the best deal on meds and pass it down to the insured.

These are the businesses that create formularies and pharmacy networks and try to streamline prescribing with programs such as e-scribing. Requiring the patient to use these formularies and programs solely would enable the PBM to monitor utilization and patient compliance with the goal of better outcomes. This has been one of the selling points to the insurers.

The "Big 3" that hold over 75% of the business are Express RX, CVS Health, and United Health OptumRX-Catamaran. There are fewer than 30 PBMs in existence today.

The PBMs make their money by getting "rebates" and adding a few percent to cover their costs. Their profits have been skyrocketing annually. These profits have been questioned so litigation is out there concerning their practices.

Today, patients are instructed by their insurance providers that they must use these PBM programs, but technically they don't have to. I think these programs have their place for the more expensive meds, but with generic and others, it pays to shop around.

My experience as a provider is that the customer service with PBMs is not so good, and many of my patients will also attest to that. This is another example — similar to the big box pharmacies and grocery stores — of potentially driving others out of the business. My gut feeling is that more of these will either get into the PBM business or start commingling so there is less competition and choice.

With such astronomical profits being questioned, along with the ethics of these PBMs, I would challenge the "Big 3" to price match. If a patient can save money on a prescription through a discount program for cash and prove it, then match it. What a concept. The grocery chains have done it for years. Why not?

Best of health!

CHAPTER 17

Prescription and Non-prescription Medications and Supplements: It Pays to Shop!

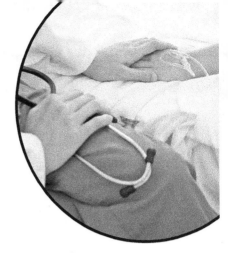

Scenario:

Christmas morning, I was spending time with my parents. My mom was eighty-nine at the time, and she shared with me that the pharmacy closest to her independent living facility told her they can charge whatever they want for over-the-counter (OTC) meds. OK, so I asked her what medication. She quickly said OTC Claritin. She takes it every three days instead of daily, as it is costing her over $1.09 per pill. That pharmacy never advised her that a generic exists. This particular pharmacy starts with the initial C and ends with an S. I was appalled as she explained what she was paying for three other OTC supplements. She was paying nearly $50 a month.

I went on Amazon and purchased 400 generic Claritin (loratadine) for $7. We also purchased the other items at 100 pills for a fraction of the cost.

This is just an example of what a markup the pharmacies choose to charge out of convenience. In my opinion this is another example of taking advantage of the elderly on a fixed income. It's just wrong.

Scenario:

In my practice, it is encouraged to electronically prescribe all meds to the preferred pharmacy on a particular insurance plan. I have heard over and over again, "My insurance requires..." I have introduced to patients the idea of shopping the insurance price vs. cash price. I had a patient who was paying around $85 for a quantity of nine generic Imitrex through the insurance. She researched options for the cash price for the same and found a deal of $18 for nine pills. She now requests written RXs (instead of electronic) for all her prescriptions. I had hundreds of patients doing the same and as a result, thousands of dollars are staying in the patients' pockets rather than the insurance. How cool is that!

Solutions:

- ✓ Shop for the best price. Protect those who aren't savvy to what's up!
- ✓ You do not have to use your insurance.
- ✓ Check out apps such as Good Rx and Blink. com for prescriptions.
- ✓ Amazon is a great source, along with big box and grocery stores, for over-the-counter medicines.

Best of health!

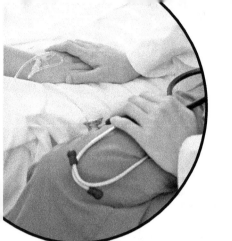

CHAPTER 18
The Opioid Epidemic

As we know, for years we in the USA have had issues with drug addiction and the costs associated with this — not only in treatment but also lack of productivity. Deaths are being reported daily due to overdose.

The buzz now is the opioid epidemic and what we are going to do about it. There is really not an easy answer. I want to share my thoughts as a healthcare provider and why this is so tough.

Years ago, "pain" became the next vital sign and we, as providers, were required to ask if a patient was in pain no matter what that person was being seen for. If you walked into a hospital room, you saw the pain scale placed on a white board with a face with frown to smiles. Providers were mandated to make sure pain was addressed at each visit.

Fast forward a few years and look at some new pain meds that have been developed. Let's take the medication Lyrica, for example. This is a great drug used for neuropathic pain and has been around since its approval by the FDA in December 2004. It was classified as a Schedule 5 controlled substance, so it has less risk for addiction. Why is it not prescribed and used more? It's all about cost. Today, after 13 years on the market, the cash price for a 30-day supply for most patients is over $400. It is still not covered by most insurers, and when it is, it is usually in the highest tier so still out-of-pocket costs can be over $100 per month through insurance.

Percocet (oxycodone) has been around since 1976 after being approved by the FDA as a Schedule 2 drug with highly addictive potential. We all know it is the go-to medication for post-surgery and has been for those with chronic pain. Now there is an urgent push to get people off these meds.

Healthcare providers' prescribing habits are under increased scrutiny as a result of these abuses. What is most concerning to me is that the cost for Oxycodone 5mg/Acetaminophen 325 mg quantity of 120 with coupon is less than $25. Need I say more, with the street value in Phoenix of over $10 a pill?

Did you know a new opioid was passed through the FDA in 2014, as it is the first extended release (24-hour) version of hydrocodone, called Hysingla? The max dose is 120 mg and comes in 40 mg tablets. The stance for this was that drug makers should concentrate on developing opioids that are harder to abuse. I am still baffled by that logic. How about we take less addictive meds such as Lyrica and make the costs of these non-controlled drugs more affordable?

I have heard of many desperate retirees on a fixed income selling their unused narcotics for food, gas, and survival. Now, think about how wrong that is on so many levels.

I know through conversations over the years that many providers would prefer not to prescribe many controlled substances. It's becoming much harder to say no to patient requests, as we are really in the middle with the pressure to provide improved patient satisfaction. Patients and even employers are following reviews such as Yelp and Health Grades to see satisfaction levels. Hospitals and practices are sending out surveys for patient satisfaction, and this data is being analyzed. These results will likely affect reimbursement for care for both providers and facilities. This is only the beginning. The ethical dilemma is doing what's right vs. "keeping patients happy"!

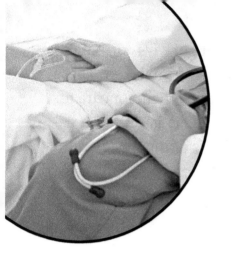

CHAPTER 19
Media: The Power of Influence— Advertising for New Medications

As a healthcare provider, I have my list of go-to medications that I have utilized over the years. Patients usually respond well and the side effect (SE) profiles are minimal. I always believed I shouldn't fix anything that is not broken.

It amazes me how patients want to jump onto the new drug bandwagon that may be indicated for their diagnoses. One watches an ad on TV that is glitzy and immediately of course it piques interest. That's the beauty of marketing and persuasion. At many appointments, people will inquire about that new drug they saw. Because of timing and curiosity, they insist on trying it. Newer is not necessarily better.

It is important to keep in mind that new medications are always very expensive. They are placed usually on the highest tier on the formulary. Because the medication is new, there is some sort of appeal that I do not understand. I would see this a lot with combination medications that would combine two generic drugs, taking one pill instead of two at a cost that was exponential.

My other concern with new medication is the record for safety and side effects. I do not want any of my patients to be the "guinea pig" for a new medication.

The safety and outcomes data will be clear once the new meds have been out for a while. Over the years, I have been fortunate to convince my patients to avoid the hype and marketing. I'm sure many of you have stories of medications you took that were pulled. Anyone remember Vioxx? It was a medication used for pain and arthritis and was pulled from the market in 2004 due to cardiac events and strokes. I remember vividly people insisting on trying it. I am glad I resisted prescribing Vioxx, as there were plenty of other options available that were proven and safer.

Unless you have a condition where there are no other medications available, my recommendation is to be patient. In time, it will become clear if a new drug is worth the cost - and more importantly, if it is safe.

Best of health!

CHAPTER 20
Saving Money:
Rebates

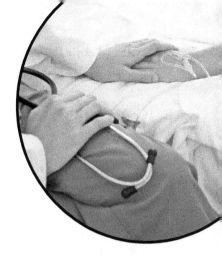

Scenario:

I was shopping over-the-counter items for my mom. I discovered she was paying so much for the convenience of her local big pharmacy — CVS — but at one huge expense.

I found a site that's brilliant. It's called Ebates. If you shop through this site, not only are you going to find the best deals, but you also get rewarded. These rebates can be upward of 10% at times.

If you are discovering that you need to work with the big pharmacies like the one that starts with a W or C, Ebates is another way to keep more money in your pocket.

Check out Ebates. The site is huge, and I am getting rebates through them for many purchases outside of health such as clothes, groceries, and travel. Let's keep more money in our pockets.

Best of health!

CHAPTER 21
Self-pay Patients—
How Do They Cope?

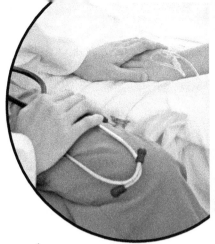

With millions of patients not having insurance, they have had to become creative and find providers that will see them. Many providers would see them and charge rates based on Medicare.

Years ago, I was working at a county clinic and the non-insured patients were being charged $120 for a visit. I remember vividly that we were disgusted that a child with strep was being charged that fee. We knew we could do it better. That was the beginning of my old practice Renaissance Family Medical Care, a rebirth of how medicine is practiced. We purposely made the decision not to accept Medicare so that we could charge a lower rate for our services. We charged a flat fee of $60 for a visit. We also were able to get discount rates at Quest and also discount x-rays and imaging through a local center in town. It worked well overall for our patients.

We could handle the preventative and also illness, but the expense came into play with specialty care! This is why I am adamant that people need to minimally have a high-deductible catastrophic policy for themselves and their families.

This is the foundation for my solution for healthcare in the US, and I continue to believe with all my heart that it will work.

Best of health!

CHAPTER 22

Impact on Losing a Business Due to a Catastrophe and No Health Insurance

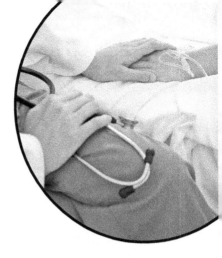

Businesses are fragile and rely on being able to function and meet expectations of their clients and employees. At any given moment, lives can change.

Scenario:

Small business owner: company with two employees. He grosses $300,000 a year. He pays employee wages but can't afford to offer health insurance. His company pays employment taxes, unemployment taxes, sales taxes, and property taxes.

This employer has a health event where he cannot work for a few months, can't pay his hospital bills, and essentially loses everything to qualify for Medicaid.

Potential effect of this:

- ✓ This is a loss of a business and a person who was contributing to employment and paying taxes.

- ✓ Employees are now unemployed and collecting income from the government as a result of unexpected life change.

- ✓ There are no longer consistent contributions from the owner, business, or employees to the tax pool. The owner's pride and dream is gone, and there is no choice but to utilize government assistance.

- ✓ This results in years of lost revenue generation for this person and family.

Solution:

This scenario for many small businesses could potentially be avoided if they had some sort of catastrophic affordable high-deductible plan. This person would have gotten care. In the meantime, potentially his business could have continued on with the help of his employees. He would have not lost his home, possibly avoided going bankrupt. Just think if that were you or a loved one!

Best of health!

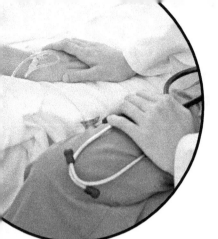

CHAPTER 23
The Healthcare Dynasties

In the last few years, whenever I thought of the healthcare giants, United Health Care was the first to come to mind, as slowly but surely they were acquiring and gaining the position of Number 1 healthcare insurer. That saddened me because the fewer the options, the less the competition, which leads to increased prices and less value. Sounds a bit like the airline industry, doesn't it?

We are used to big systems like Kaiser and Cigna that are essentially all in one "doc in the box." Within their organizations are providers, specialists, ancillary, pharmacies, and X-ray...but usually no hospitals.

Now we are seeing huge mergers: CVS and Aetna. Think about it...they have the health plan and pharmacy piece, but other than their CVS Minute

Clinics, not the provider piece. I doubt CVS will be exclusive to Aetna, so they potentially will continue to be a big player in the pharmacy piece that all the insurance companies negotiate with.

An important question to ponder is why there may be conflict of interest with this merger.

There are rumblings that the mega-giant Walmart is positioning itself to acquire Humana. Amazon is now seriously considering entering the pharmaceutical business, just like they did with the food industry with the recent acquisition of Whole Foods.

Times are really changing! It is going to be fascinating to wait and see if healthcare costs go down long term and if any savings are passed to the consumer.

Time will tell. Just sit back and think about how these potential and closed acquisitions will affect you and your family.

I am still trying to absorb the potential for greater profits that all these players are going to have. My prediction is their management and stockholders are going to be very happy!...But at whose expense?

Best of health!

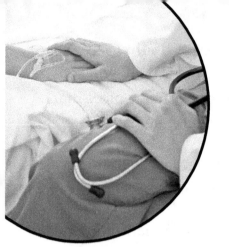

CHAPTER 24
Healthcare for Profit:
Awesome Times for
Stockholders and
CEOs

Affordable Health Care became effective in March 2010. We all should be aware that the goal was to provide affordable care for all and bring down costs.

This has also been a period in history where the insurance companies have had extraordinary profits for the stockholders and CEOs.

Company	January 2009	September 2018
United	$26.50 per share Value of 1,000 shares = **$26,500**	$265.30 per share Value of 1,000 shares = **$265,300**
Cigna	$16.00 per share Value of 1,000 shares = **$16,000**	$195.00 per share Value of 1,000 shares = **$195,000**
Aetna	$23.80 per share Value of 1,000 shares = **$23,800**	$202.75 per share Value of 1,000 shares = **$202,750**

I wish I had gotten even a few shares...over nine years we are looking at 800-1000% profits.

The pharmacies did very well, but nothing like what we see with the insurance:

Company	January 2009	September 2018
CVS	$25.75 per share Value of 1,000 shares = **$25,750**	$76.91 per share Value of 1,000 shares = **$76,910**
Walgreens	$25.50 per share Value of 1,000 shares = **$25,500**	$70.20 per share Value of 1,000 shares = **$70,200**

Still, over 250% profits. Not bad.

At the same time, CEO salaries and bonuses grew along with trends...

Check these numbers that were reported for 2016:

Company	Salary
United	$14.5 million with total compensation of $31.3 million
Cigna	$15.2 million with total compensation of $49.0 million
Aetna	$18.6 million with total compensation of $27.9 million
CVS	$18.5 million
Walgreens	$13.7 million

The average CEO salary in the USA is $760,000

Sit back and try to absorb this...why such profits after the Affordable Care Act (ACA)?

Some thoughts to ponder:

If you, as a private investor, invested in these stocks, you would be sitting in a very comfortable position. Huge profits were realized in a short period of time.

Unfortunately, these gains were at the patients', providers', and facilities' expense. Patient premiums continue to rise, and provider/facility reimbursements have been essentially flat.

The insurance companies have continued to withdraw from the exchanges, because apparently they were not making enough money. At least, that was one of the excuses they gave.

There were no penalties outlined by the government for insurance companies if they pulled out of the ACA.

This is a lot of information to take in and absorb, but maybe you should? Everyone, politics aside, should at least agree that these results really swayed away from the original intent of affordable care for all. At least, I think so!

Best of health!

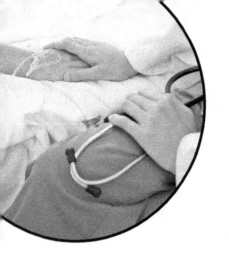

CHAPTER 25

My Solution for Providing Healthcare for All in the USA, and I Am Sticking with It.

This was a letter I wrote in 2008 and sent to our Congress and presidential candidates. The same letter with minimal changes was again hand delivered to a local congresswoman in the summer of 2017. The content has essentially stayed the same.

Dear K.S.,

It was a pleasure to meet you today, and I really look forward to what can be accomplished in the next few years. Many people are very nervous about the future, and this is to be expected. I so hope that Congress and President–Elect Trump can find common ground and truly make a positive impact on all Americans.

As I stated, after being in family practice and owning my own medical practice, I have heard over and over the same theme from my patients, family, and friends. People are worried about the medical catastrophic event that could wipe out their family's savings in hours. Many have shared with me their stories, fears, and willingness to pay into a system to provide such coverage. It pains everyone to hear proposed solutions leading to more cuts and higher out-of-pocket expenses in programs that people have contributed to as part of their taxation since entering the work force. I feel strongly that we can shore up existing programs such as Medicare and also provide care for those when they need it the most.

Solution 1: Immediately rid the billing practice of "usual and customary" rates. As you know, these rates are inflated and unrealistic. I propose that if you are a tax-paying citizen in this country, have no health insurance and end up at a hospital, doctor's office or ancillary facility, you are billed at a rate that is about 100%-120% of Medicare, rather than the highly inflated "usual and customary" rates.

Solution 2: MY Grand Plan: Catastrophic insurance for all those who cannot qualify for insurance in the traditional ways. We take a system that is already in place - Medicare - and we extend it out to the 27-40 million people with no coverage. We do a cost analysis and charge a fair premium and determine a deductible that is based on income and other parameters to be determined.

Obama Care has struggled because there were too many loopholes that allowed the private insurers to bail out. They were not committed — as we all know, it's about profit and performance of their stocks. I think the intention was amazing but there was no way this 2,000-page bill could be executed.

My patients are outraged that the only choice they now have in Maricopa County is Ambetter. Not many providers take it, and even if people can afford to pay the ridiculously high premiums, they still will not get the care they need. I could go on and on. If Congress could first focus on ensuring every American has a catastrophic plan, I truly believe we will see less bankruptcies and financial ruin, and at the same time Medicare could become more solvent and self-sustaining for future generations.

Sincerely,

Barbara G Regis, MS PA-C
Ask the PA: Your Healthcare Advocate.
Bgregis@cox.net

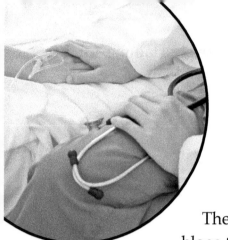

CHAPTER 26
Physician Satisfaction

There are a lot of articles and blogs that discuss physician dissatisfaction with their jobs. Many people continue to feel doctors make too much money. We all can agree with the notion that they do make a very decent wage; however, the amount of time to get the degree can be mindboggling.

For a family practice provider, there is an 11-year minimum commitment, being 4 years for undergrad, 4 years for medical school, and 3 years residency. Surgeons and other specialists can continue on for a few more years after that. Many end up with student loans in the $200,000-300,000 range. So out of the starting gate there are hundreds of thousands of dollars in student debt, plus unrecognized income from not being able to work. Some students, if they do not strike a deal to work for a few years in underserved communities, have student loan payments in the $3,000-4,000 a month range for 15-20 years.

The average family physician salary is $195,000 compared to $284,000 for other specialties. This is a reason many physicians are electing to go into other fields of medicine, which contributes to the shortage of primary physicians. For those who are in the field, there are increased workloads.

A solution is making medical education more afford-able and providing incentives for those who commit to primary care. Do not be fooled into thinking that all physicians are "rich." It just is not the case.

As we continue to have physician shortages, it is predicted that in 2025 there will be a shortage of 12,000-31,000 physicians. As PAs we are helping with the shortfall but even then, it does not come close to being at an acceptable level.

It is time to open more slots and make sure that the right people are getting in. It is not just about test scores, but passion and dedication to the profes-sion. It is a calling, whether you agree or not.

Best of health!

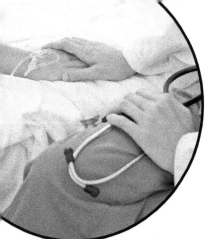

CHAPTER 27
The Legal Side of Healthcare

Medical Malpractice:

This is a discussion that is difficult because depending on where you live, it can have a huge impact on healthcare and the associated costs.

Let's look at it from the viewpoints of some of the players involved.

1. The patient: there is no doubt that when there is a huge mistake, it will affect you for the rest of your life. It's the legitimate claims vs. the waste of time claims. Providers are human, and all of us can look back at a situation that could have been handled better, but do you need to have a claim?

2. Providers have insurance but in today's world of medicine many have become very

defensive and will do almost anything to keep a patient happy. This leads to sometimes additional testing and also writing prescriptions that may not necessarily be in the best interest of the patient.

3. Hospitals are subject to claims involving any service they offer from the time the patient arrives at the doorstep until that individual is back home after being discharged.

4. Lawyers want business. Some work for the provider but many more for the patient. All the advertising: "Have you ever experienced..." and you know the rest. We all know many in politics are lawyers, and they have no incentive to pass reforms that affect them and their fellow attorneys' bottom lines.

Tort Reform:

There has been a push to place caps/limits on the amount of money patients can receive on malpractice claims federally, but Congress has not yet passed any legislation to limit claim payouts and punitive damages on a federal level.

Thirty-three states have passed reforms to try to bring down costs and decrease frivolous suits. As a result, more providers are going to consider practicing in those states. These reforms have a huge impact on costs and provider longevity. Think about it...supply and demand because more providers practice there, decreased costs for malpractice insurance, provider satisfaction - and hopefully this would affect premiums as well.

Did you know that if you get your care through the federal government such as the VA and Indian Health Service, it is more difficult to resolve a claim, and it is very expensive and time-consuming? Because providers are federal employees, they are not required to have malpractice insurance. In the VA and IHS, these claims are addressed only through federal courts after a waiting period. This is a result of the Federal Tort Claims Act of 1946.

Healthcare Costs and Unnecessary Testing:

Did you know that in the US in 2016 around $200 billion was spent in performing tests that may not have been necessary? On top of this, some procedures led to around 30,000 deaths.

So why is this happening? My mom would say it so eloquently: "They are covering their butt." Well, she has a point.

What I love about practicing cradle to grave is that I have had the best elderly patients. We would get into the discussion about what they wanted ultimately for their health and recommendations that made sense for them. There are unfortunately providers out there who don't or won't have these conversations, out of fear or unwillingness to think logically about what makes sense for each patient.

Let's give some examples:

1. Ordering a mammogram on a 75-year-old with no previous history of abnormal results, who does not want the test anymore.

2. How about a PSA on an 85-year-old who has no history or symptoms?

3. Or a colonoscopy on an 80-year-old with no family history.

4. In the ER, performing repeat testing with utilization of standing orders.

These are examples that drive up costs. If I have an extremely healthy 75-year-old with concerns and wants to be worked up, exceptions should be considered when it comes to testing. I have seen amazingly healthy people that age who were diagnosed with very early cancers and in remission while still enjoying active lives today.

The question to consider when working up an older patient is very simple. What are we going to do with those results? If nothing, don't go there.

Another problem seen too frequently is repeating the same tests by multiple providers. In primary care, if a diagnosis presents that will require surgery, I will punt to the appropriate surgical specialty with a workup. Testing and scans may have been ordered but many times, especially in the ER, they repeat those studies again anyway. Hospitals seem to be incentivized to test over and over.

One of the goals with electronic medical records (EMRs) is creating the ability for healthcare providers and facilities to communicate with each other. The development and utilization of patient portals will help the patients' ability to access their records. This piece alone should hopefully help decrease unnecessary testing. Time will tell. As a patient and family member, having speedy access to health information excites me. Simple steps like this should not only lead to better outcomes, but also can save money leading to decreased costs.

Perspective for providers: Places to work and costs of malpractice insurance

Medscape released its survey on the best and worst places to practice medicine and it was a bit of a shock.

Best places:

1. Minneapolis, MN
2. Madison, WI
3. Sioux Falls, ID
4. Des Moines, IA
5. Burlington, VT
6. Boston, MA

The attraction was a combination of high employer-sponsored insurance, healthier population, lower malpractice suits, and better collaboration among providers.

The worst places to practice were a surprise to me, as Phoenix was second to New Orleans:

1. New Orleans, LA
2. Phoenix, AZ
3. Las Vegas, NV
4. Albuquerque, NM
5. Tulsa, OK

Dissatisfaction in New Orleans: High malpractice cases and also poorer populations and less employer-sponsored insurance. All have some form of tort reform, except Arizona.

Here are a few examples of malpractice premiums. You will easily see who has reform and who doesn't:

Specialty	State	Malpractice Premium
Internal Medicine	Florida	$47,707
	New York	$37,877
	California	$4,168
	Nebraska	$2,810
General Surgery	Florida	$190,926
	New York	$141,608
	California	$16,982
	Nebraska	$9,552
OB/GYN	New York	$195,891
	California	$16,240

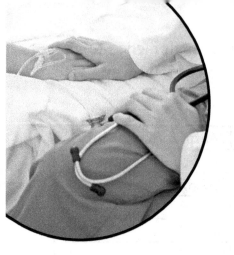

CHAPTER 28
Healthcare:
Yesterday, Today
and Tomorrow...

As you can see, healthcare in my dad's day was much more hands-on and not as much accessibility to tests and labs...it was so much more based on history, physical exam, experience, and then the appropriate intervention. Think of it... back then the imaging available was limited to x-rays and ultrasound.

MRI technology was not available to the mainstream until the early '80s, as it received approval for medical use in the mid-'70s. Then finally the first body scanner was produced. Prior to that, people relied on either the physician's office for simple labs or the local hospital for more extensive labs and imaging.

It was not until the late '60s when Quest labs opened its first lab for business, followed a few years later by Lab Corp.

The first ambulances as we know them were established in the 1960s. My father saw the evolution of all this during his first years of practice.

Today we have evolved to a more sophisticated model, with Electronic Medical Records (EMRs), labs and x-rays, as well as pharmacies being more accessible. There is much more competition and choice. Medicine is still being practiced in the brick and mortar and also through telemedicine. The goals continue to be more consumer-oriented.

Now we are continuing to evolve, with the addition of sophisticated tools that monitor your blood pressure, glucose, exercise, and nutrition. There are health coaches assigned to help you become healthier. Continuous monitoring devices are not only beneficial to the patient, but also to the provider to predict outcomes as well as improve efficiencies.

We are now in the age of stem cell research, genetic engineering, and 3D imaging. These applications to the practice of medicine will be mind-boggling.

The question we will have to ask is whether all of these new technologies are truly an adjunct part of care, or in time could they potentially replace the one-on-one patient/provider experience?

The world of medicine is changing rapidly, as our world demands this through advances in technology.

It will ultimately come down to outcomes and what you, the patient, expect and demand.

Time will tell. Best of health!

CHAPTER 29
Final Thoughts on the Financial Side of Healthcare

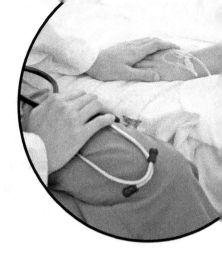

My goal with this book has simply been to introduce the idea of changing the way we think about our health, and I hope to get constructive conversations going. I truly feel we are at a pivotal time. I am concerned about the direction we are headed, and as I chat with many people, I know I am not alone.

It is time to iron out the fundamental question concerning healthcare as a privilege or right. We should be able to agree that everyone during his or her life will require some form of medical care. Given this, it is not a choice but honestly a necessity for all.

With the mergers of CVS and Aetna, possibly Walmart and Humana, and the mergers of United with large physician groups, we are seeing a lot of co-mingling of different interests in the healthcare equation. Sit back and think about where this is going and who will be left out in the dust.

I really feel that medicine as my father knows it and I know it will continue to become a lost art/ profession. The relationship between the patient and provider will become more dictated through many outside factors, with the goal of pure profit. As we can see, this is already happening.

It's going to be very interesting to see ultimately where this country continues to go with the "business of healthcare." I hope we can get serious dialogue going. Just sayin'!

Best of health!

About Barb

Prior to becoming a Physician Assistant (PA), Barb was an accomplished musician and teacher. She holds dual bachelor's degrees from Arizona State University in Education and Music Performance, with her main instrument being the euphonium. She performed locally and taught band to students at Madison Meadows School upon graduation.

In 1992, Barb made the conscious decision to leave teaching and her musical career in pursuit of a career in medicine. She worked for two years at Maricopa Medical Center, assigned to the burn center, where she developed a new level of understanding of patient care and teamwork. At that time, she attended ASU and Grand Canyon University, obtaining her prerequisites for furthering her education.

She was accepted into AT Still University's first PA class in 1995 and graduated in 1997 with a Master's of Science in Physician Assistant Studies. Since graduation, she has worked in family practice. She spent her first five years working at several Maricopa County outpatient clinics in the Phoenix area.

She then had the opportunity to become a partner in Renaissance Medical Group and Renaissance Medical Properties in Chandler and Maricopa, Arizona. For the next fourteen years, she had a dual role of chief operations officer and practicing PA.

As a result of being in charge of day-to-day operations and human resources at Renaissance, she has gained significant knowledge concerning the business side of medicine. During that time, she also gained hands-on experience working with architects and contractors, designing and opening up three new offices.

She also has been adjunct professor for Northern Arizona University's PA program and has precepted PA students as well as third and fourth year medical students through the years.

After leaving Renaissance, she worked for One Medical Group as a PA but also on-boarded providers and practices locally and nationally with the Practice Integration Team based in San Francisco.

She is currently working for Premise Health at Insight Enterprises in Tempe, Arizona as a solo practitioner/health center manager, providing primary care to employees and families on campus.

She is certified by the National Commission of Certification of Physician Assistants and is a fellow member of the American Academy of Physician Assistants.

She loves advocating for patients, families, and health providers, as she is very active through social media with her Facebook page ASK THE PA. She also recently has become involved in melanoma awareness/support.

She also enjoys hosting and highlighting the passions of great practitioners, advocates, and patients through her radio show *Best of Health* at Phoenix Business Radio X.

In her spare time, she loves to travel, maintaining an active lifestyle that includes running, biking, swimming. She loves to spend time outdoors with her husband Tony, family and friends, whether it's walking on the beach or hiking in the desert. Sunscreen and UV protective attire are her new best friends.

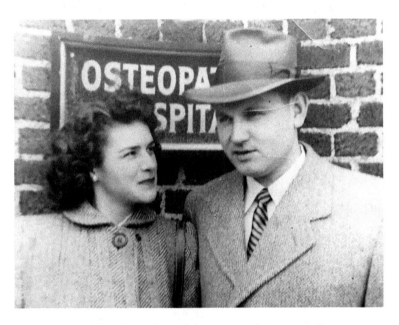

Mom and Dad ready to start their practice

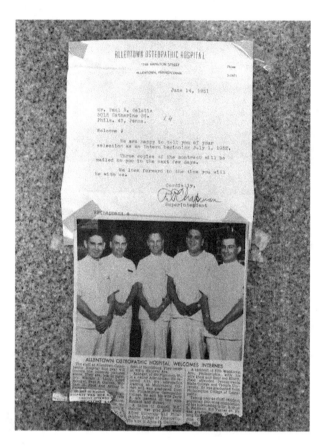

Dad's Residency Graduation

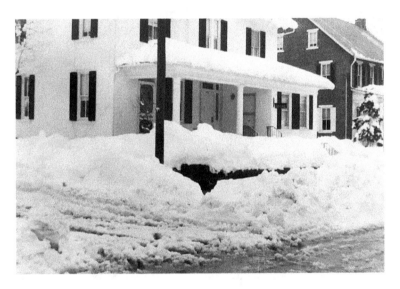

House Office on Main St

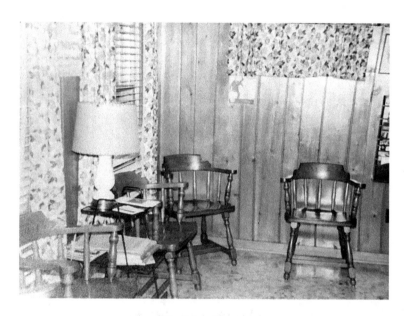

Waiting Room

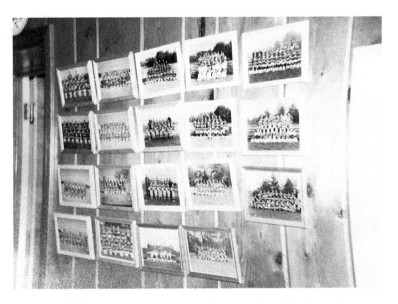

Team Dr. for many teams displayed in Dad's office

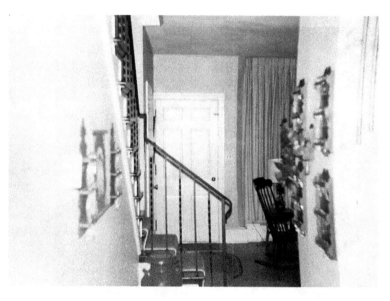

The front door to our home and reception area for guests

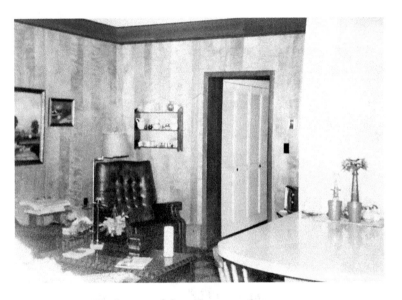

Kitchen and family room bar area...
lots of interesting conversations took place here

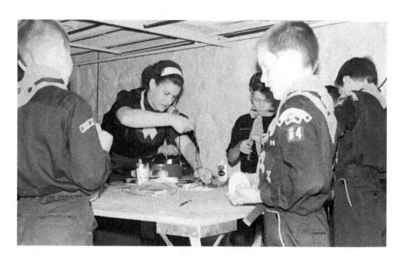

Mom, Dave and her scouting troop

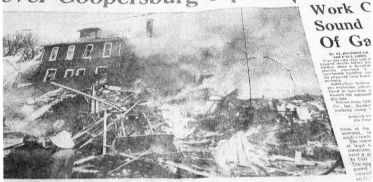

The morning paper

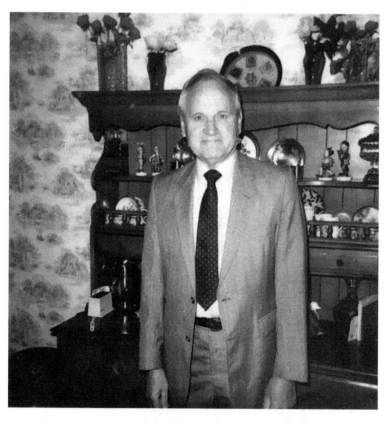

Dad dressed up for Recognition event after explosion

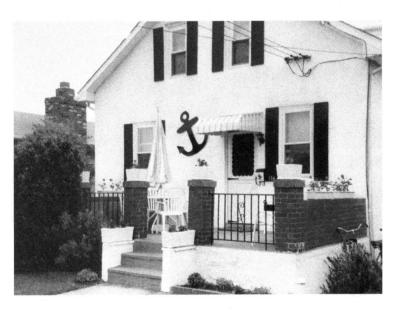

The Shore house...our family escape

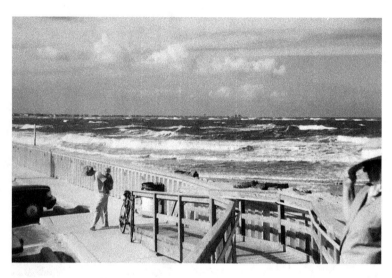

Avalon - Atlantic Ocean near our place

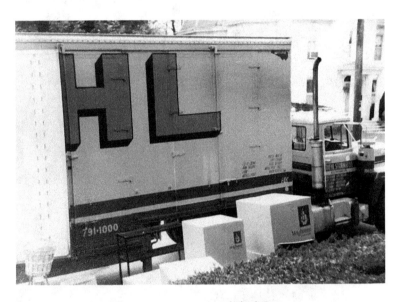

Moving Day - on to a new life for my parents

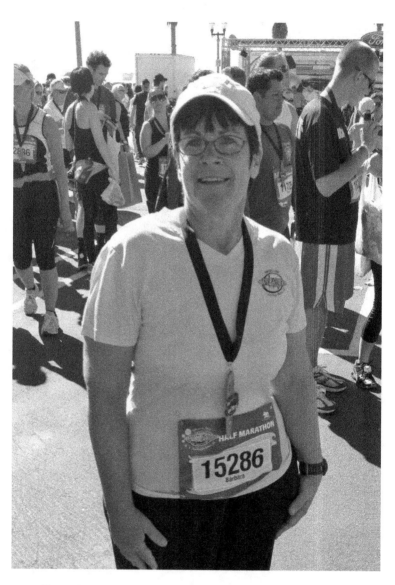

Running...my passion and happy place pre-cancer

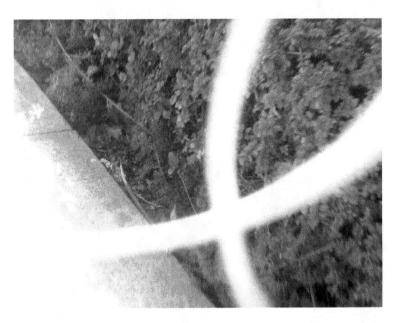

Running and this was on my phone...
Melanoma warrior and fighter

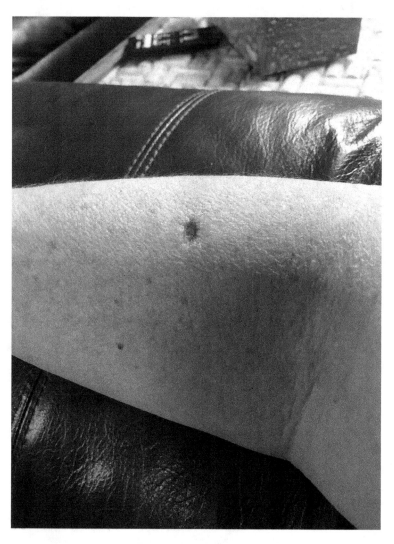

Biopsy site...nodular Melanoma

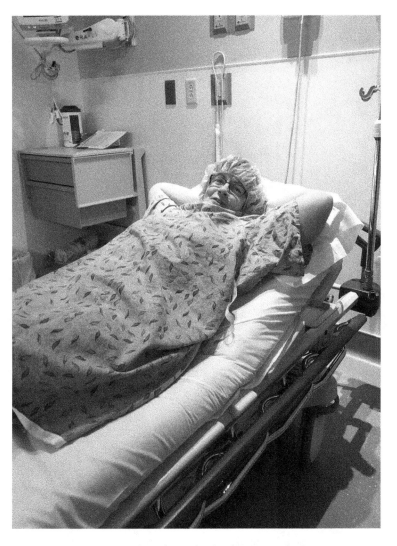

Prepped and ready for surgery and
sentinel lymph node biopsy (SLNB)

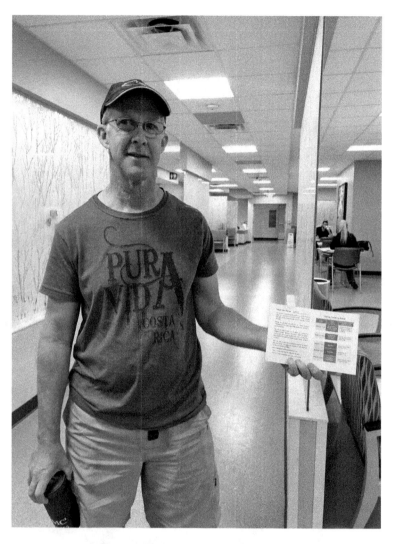

My surgery day...Tony's tracking monitor

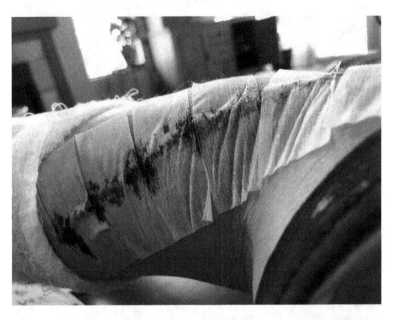

Wide excision and round 2 goes to ME!

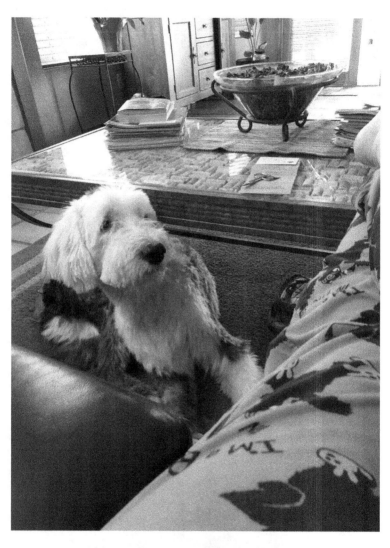

Abby making sure I rest and recover

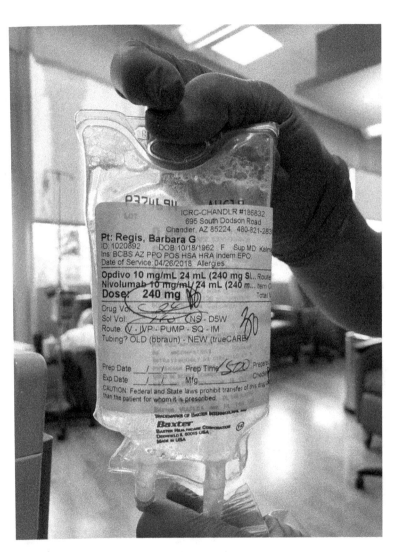

Immunotherapy-Opdivo

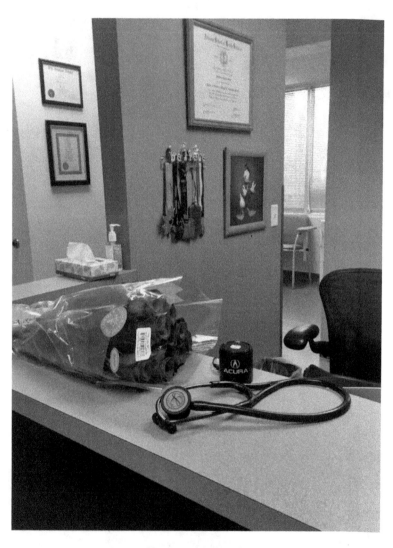

My office and being loved...

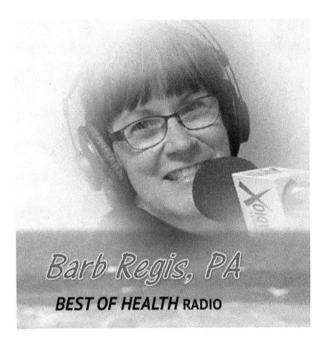

Barb Regis, PA
BEST OF HEALTH RADIO

Sharing great people and stories
Your Health, Your Business

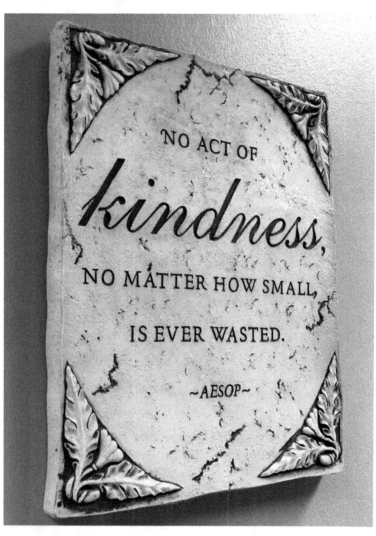

My Mantra

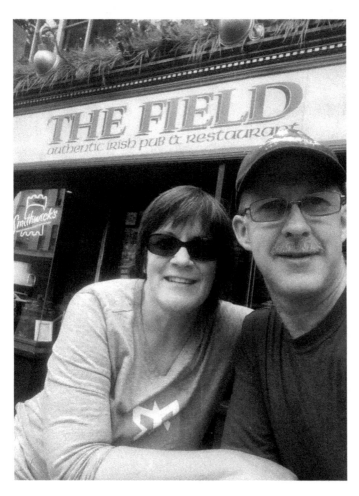

Tony and I loving life

CPSIA information can be obtained
at www.ICGtesting.com
Printed in the USA
FSHW020308011220